Kiss Me Again!

7 Secrets To Kisses That Drive Her Wild!

By

Mike Johnson

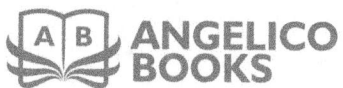

TABLE OF CONTENTS

CHAPTER 1

Overview

Become an amazing kisser and ignite her passions for more!

Did you know that the brain is our biggest sex organ?

Did you know that a recent study found that how well you kiss can be the make or break to whether a woman even considers having sex with you?

Did you know that recent research shows that women evaluate how good a lover a man will be by his kissing?

You're probably already a good kisser, and maybe you've read some books on kissing. That's great!

But you might be picking up this book because:

1. You're new to kissing and you want to develop the confidence to do it well, and learn the tips and tricks to avoid rejection.

2. You want to spice up your kissing life. You're a

great kisser but you realize that most couples get into a 'kissing rut' and you want to learn new kissing techniques to try out with your partner.

3. You aren't getting the reaction that you want from your kisses, so you want to get better so you get more.

Here is your opportunity to learn the 'world-class kissing secrets that only a handful of lucky people knew existed a short time ago, including step-by-step skills, know-how and techniques of:

1. Guaranteeing that your partner has an amazing experience every time you kiss her.

2. How to NEVER get rejected again when you want to kiss a girl!

3. You'll get step-by-step proven kissing techniques that will make you the leader of the kissing pack.

And that's just a taste of what you'll find in this short but information-packed book!

Here's the thing. You already know the basics. You can find them on the Internet. What we add is the breakthrough information that will take you to the next level – or get you started right!

Now is the time to take action. At this time in our society, we need more connection and great sizzle. The people I know are feeling more and more disconnected, the art of love has gone way out of style, and we need to bring it back. And you can!

The only way you are ever going to do that is to read this book from cover to cover, and take action.

When you do, you'll find that you are the person the girls flock around, and the other men and boys will be asking you your secrets.

You'll learn (as I did) that when you are an amazing kisser, you can:

- Have a fantastic kiss (and even more) before the first date is even over!

- Build the confidence to ask any girl out and have her say yes!

- Have the girls asking you out and making the first moves!

Of course most people don't pick up a book like this. They don't think they have what it takes. They feel like they are too young, or too old, or too nervous, or too inexperienced to learn how to do this.

WRONG!

Anyone who can communicate can learn to be an amazing kisser! The reasons people go wrong is because they don't know how. They don't have a system.

Well, in buying this book, you now have a system. We'll take you by the hand, step-by-step and teach you:

- what she's thinking

- types of kissing

- how to make the approach (and never get rejected again)

- how to French kiss

- secrets to making her come back for more

How do I know this?

I used to be clueless. I was too scared to make the first move on a date, and when I did try to kiss a girl, it turned out horribly. Remember all those nerdy failures in the movies? That was me, only worse.

Then I ran into this guy named Eban, a short, skinny geeky guy who had the touch of gold. Within a week of being in town he had all the most beautiful women around him. So, being desperate, I shook off my pride and begged him to teach me what he knew. After three weeks of groveling, he finally took pity on me, and in one afternoon taught me the primary secrets that you're going to read today. It's that simple.

Within a week my confidence was up, I asked a couple of girls out, and I tried these amazing techniques. And they worked! Since then I've added to what I've learned, and honed it down into this short, easy-to-read manual on how to kiss a girl.

Read it, and go out and put it into practice. You'll be amazed what a difference it makes!

So, let's start by busting some myths about kissing:

Myth 1: Amazing kissing is all about flowery poetry and romance. NOT TRUE. I've had amazing kisses in a parking lot with someone I've just met. Now, if at first you don't have a whole lot of confidence and ability to connect, then romance is key. Studies show that girls are more turned on in quiet romantic settings, so you up your chances of success when you set a romantic mood.

Myth 2: Kissing is an art, you can't learn it from a book. NOT TRUE. Of course practicing improves your skills, but kissing is a skill, like driving or walking. At first you might not be confident at it, and that's why you have this book to jumpstart your knowledge and skills!

Myth 3: Trying to kiss a girl can get you rejected. NOT TRUE. When you follow the first kiss program we have in this book, you will NEVER be rejected again when you kiss a girl. So, read on and learn!

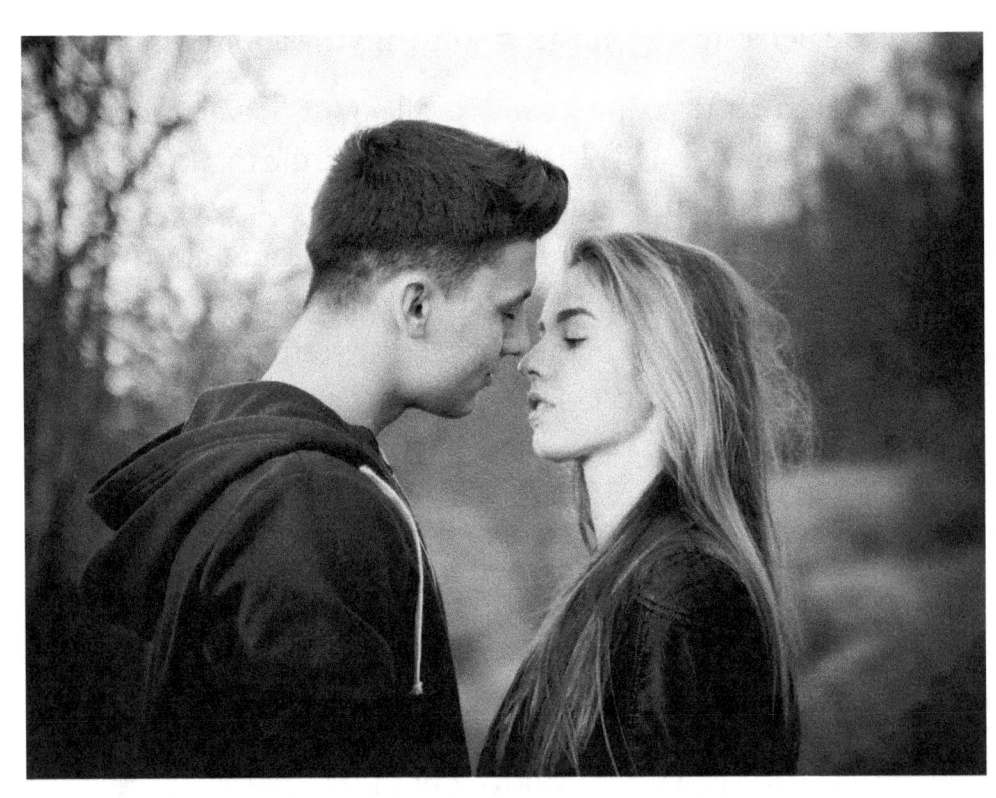

CHAPTER 2

7 Steps to Being a Master Kisser

During this instruction you'll learn everything you need to become a master kisser.

Here's what you can expect:

1. *Understand What's Going On In Her Head:* First we'll take you deep into her mind. To understand how to kiss a girl, it helps to understand what's going on in her head before, during and after you kiss her so you'll know how to approach the situation.

2. *Know Your Kissing Styles:* You'll learn all about the different types of kissing styles and how to choose the right one for the occasion. You may have some doubts about your ability to kiss and may even feel awkward when in a close with a girl. Not to worry, we're here to provide you with everything you need to know to become the kisser that the girls talk about with those secret smiles. You'll also read true stories that will help explain nearly

everything you need to know to learn about how a woman thinks, what you should and shouldn't do and how to really understand the intricacies of what she means by paying attention to the right details.

3. *Learn the French Kiss:* After learning about different types of kissing, we focus in on the most magical (and most powerful) French kiss. We'll tell you all about it and how to do it right and have her coming back for more. You'll also learn all of the important dos and don'ts for this masterful style.

4. *Make the First Kiss Special:* If you're just starting to date, the all-important first kiss will be discussed so you can get off on the right foot. This kiss is the most important and has a lot of rules to go along with it. We'll make sure you have everything in your arsenal available to make it special.

5. *Bad Kissing vs. Good Kissing:* The good, the bad and the ugly. Find out what not to do so you avoid turning her off, and what you should do so she'll see stars. You'll be surprised at how much information you'll learn from one simple book that will make a big difference in her life. We'll also get you to the point where you can be considered a master kisser with the extra details you'll need to drive her wild. There are a lot of subtle things

you can do that have nothing to do with kissing that can make all the difference in the world.

6. *Teach Her to be a Kissing Master:* What if she's not a good kisser? We'll show you how you can teach her to kiss better without her ever knowing!

7. *Advanced Topics:* We'll teach you the secret techniques to make you irresistible so she won't be able to get enough of you. There are so many things you can do to make your kiss above and beyond what she's ever experienced before.

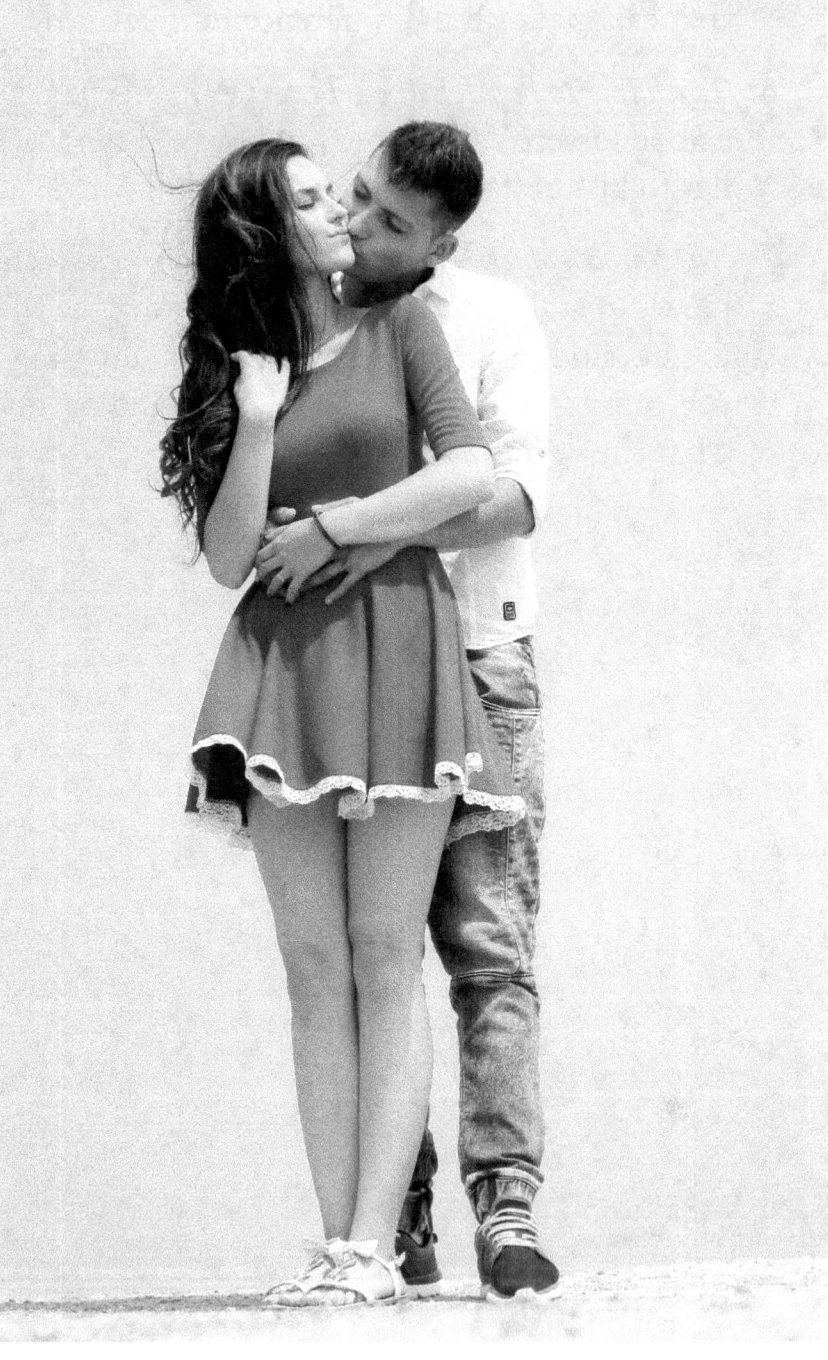

CHAPTER 3

Understand What's Going On in Her Head

Men and women are different. No matter what you think or believe, there's no denying that a kiss can make you weak in the knees or make you run for the next woman. But it's even more important for the girl! Yes, we love to kiss and it can make us like a girl even more, but face it, we guys could skip the kiss and get right down to business.

For women, it's completely different. Studies show that a 'bad' kisser will completely turn a woman off and she may decide right then and there that you aren't the one for her. Forget sex at that point – she's already made up her mind and there's no turning back. So getting the first kiss right is critical. That's why we wrote this book!

The Science of Kissing

The big question – why do we kiss? Really, think about it. It's strange how something so simple can make such a big difference. From a biological point of view, kissing releases a rush of brainwave messages, chemicals, scents and emotions. It increases feelings of closeness and bonding (especially in the girl), and of course increases sexual desire. I'm not going to bore you with the latest research, but I will say this – kissing can't be explained scientifically, yet there are a lot of theories that make a lot of sense.

It's important to give you a little insight into what happens during a kiss as far as your body and mind are concerned, as well as a little history about how the kiss came about and what turned it into what it is today. This background knowledge will help give you a deeper understanding and provide you with the core knowledge you need to start your journey.

Some say the concept of kissing began when a mother passed food to her child using her mouth, thus creating a bond between them.

Others say kissing is completely chemical, that males pass testosterone to the female, relaxing her and getting her in the mood. Reportedly, the more you kiss, the more she'll get in the mood and increase her desire to have sex.

There's also the theory that kissing is a way for the man and woman to chemically 'check each other out' and see if they would create healthy children. This theory suggests we may be assessing our date for potential diseases, health and our biological compatibility, all through the information we pick up from a kiss

Pheromones, or chemical 'smells' that can't necessarily be detected by the average human, have been linked to desire and interest in another person. Your senses will pick them up without you even giving it a thought. Even though there's no concrete proof of how it works, scientists accept the fact that pheromones do exist and probably alter our behavior. It's known to work for some animals because they have receptive organs that determine the scent of potential mates, but studies on humans haven't been quite so conclusive. Still, we're all animals, right?

Bonding

Kissing isn't just an act in and of itself; it's an emotional bonding event that takes place between people who have formed a connection. The phrase, 'the kiss that made the world stop', isn't all that far from reality. When you kiss a woman, it's just the two of you and you're completely focused only on that person. You may completely lose all sense of the world and others around you. This is especially true for women. In order for the kiss to happen, both individuals must have some connection and be willing to let their guard down and completely trust one another. Curiosity and anticipation abounds. You're exploring each other to see what it's like to truly be intimate with them before sex even becomes a possibility. For the first kiss, this is at the core of what's involved. Every other kiss that follows may never live up to that first one, and you'll always remember it!

The History of Kissing

So where did kissing come from and when did it begin? Glad you asked. The earliest known depiction of kissing goes back to 1500 B.C. It was discovered in Hindu writings found in India. Although there's nothing concrete that shows acts of kissing, there are references to using the tongue and lips. The Babylonians were also known to depict kissing on stone tablets. Most of them only showed kissing as a way to greet someone. The first writings to explore   the act of kissing come from the Kama Sutra, and there are plenty of references to kissing in that book.

The most controversial discussion of kissing comes from the Christian tradition. The Bible contains many examples of kissing, both for showing respect to elders and in acts of love. The church was extremely worried about what kissing would lead to. They even went as far as creating laws in order to keep their parishioners from committing carnal sin. This even led to the segregation of the sexes.

The Greeks have plenty of references to kissing in many forms of literature. They talk about kissing as a means to show respect and other writings show kissing as part of a courtship between man and woman. More references to the act of kissing can be found in the writings and art of nearly every early culture, including the Persians, Ethiopians and Egyptians.

The culture with the most writings about kissing is probably the ancient Romans. Not only did they depict kissing in a lot of their stories, kissing came in all forms for them – romantic and social, physical and nonphysical. So much so that they were considered to be the ones that introduced kissing to all of the new cultures they met. The Romans made kissing an art form, and reportedly made mouth-to-mouth kissing popular around the world.

Kissing was also a way of confirming deals as a 'visual' way of sealing contracts. Since many people were illiterate thousands of years ago, they were unable to read or sign documents to seal the deal. Thus the saying "sealed with a kiss" and the use of the X as a signature began. Back then, kissing was also a way of showing your status among others and it's even used in some forms today. Think about royalty or the Pope. Many will kiss the ring, hand or robe of royalty or church leaders to show their loyalty and respect. It was very common back then and often a requirement for those who to met the visiting kings and queens.

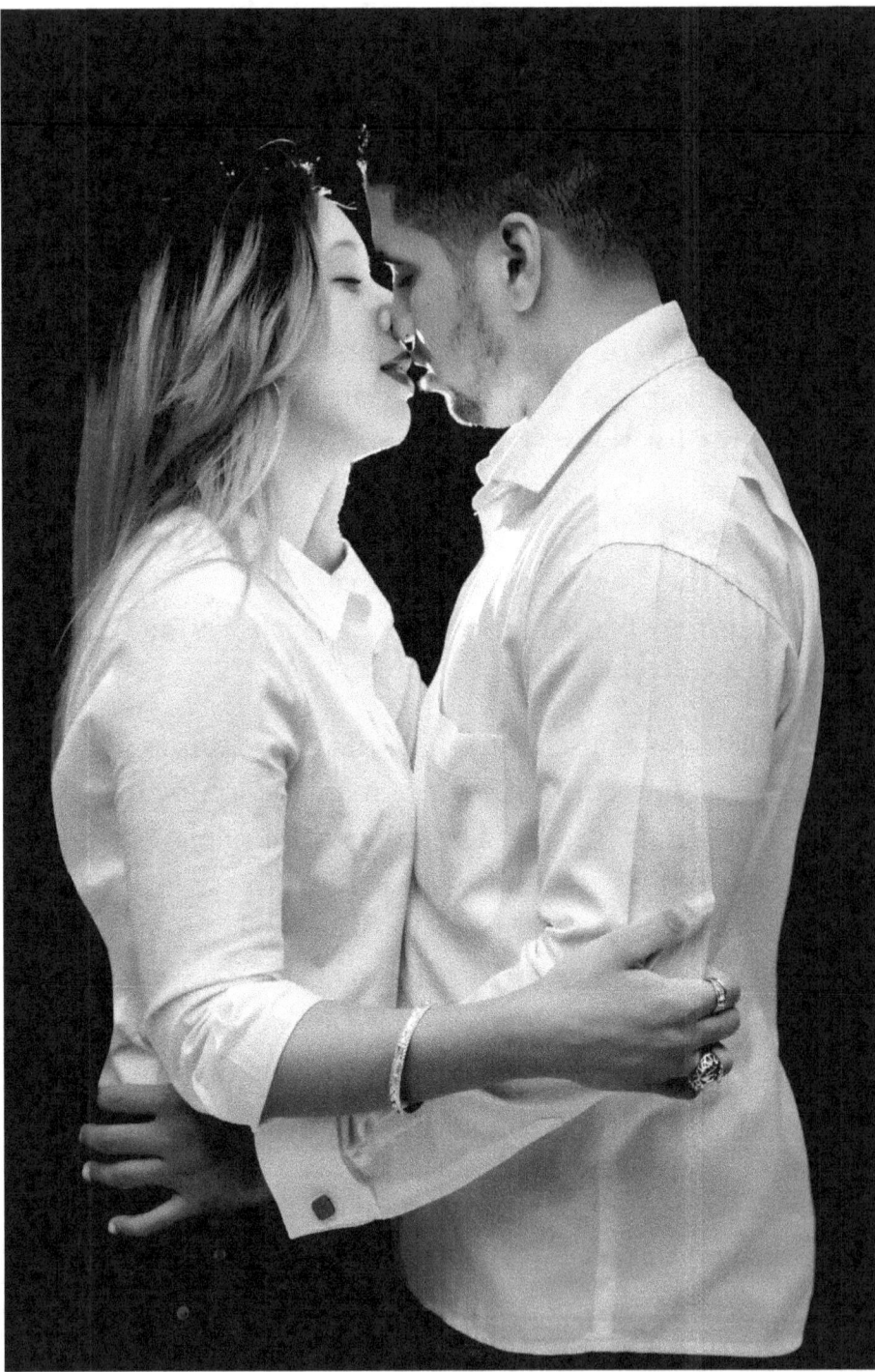

CHAPTER 4

Know the 12 Kissing Styles

I get this question a lot: "What type of kiss should it be?" There are a lot more styles than you probably know, but your best bet is to understand the situation first. If it's your first kiss ever, you'll probably want to stick with the peck. We're not talking about a peck on the cheek here – this is where you can start to become more intimate, starting with a peck on the lips.

A Peck: The peck is a closed-mouth quick smooch. Lips are soft, dry and closed. Generally lasts between less than a second to three seconds.

However, it depends on how long you've known the girl and what your standing is with her. If you've known her quite some time and you're moving from friends into a more involved relationship, you probably want to give her the more romantic sensual kiss with your lips slightly parted. Otherwise she might get the idea that you're just trying to remain friends.

If you're ending a first date, you want it to be something between a peck and a passionate kiss. If you are just looking to be a better kisser with the partner you already have, the following are some great ideas:

- *Simple kiss:* a gentle meeting of the lips. The lips are soft, relaxed. This is especially nice done slowly with a gentle move in. Also, the more feeling you put into this one, the more romance it has. The key is soft, dry lips.

- *Sensual or Soft Kiss:* a soft kiss that lasts longer than a peck or simple kiss. Again, soft lips, slightly parted (enough that you could hold a pencil in your mouth) and gently meet her lips with a little more pressure than the simple kiss. It's best to choose her upper or lower lip to place yours around so that one of your lips is between hers and visa versa. To make this one a little longer, gently and slowly allow your lips to kiss different parts of her mouth.

- *Teaser:* gently nibble on her lip and let go. This isn't actually a kiss per se; it's more of a prelude for the real kiss to come. This is a short 'kiss', almost like the peck only a different version. The nibble should be soft, and you can add to it by looking into her eyes and giving her a teasing smile.

- *Swirl and press:* touch her lips lightly with yours, and then swirl your tongue around and enter deeper into her mouth. Some girls love this, so it's always good to give it a shot.

- *French kiss:* using your tongue to play with hers. This kiss can be used like the teaser for a short period of time, the all-out kiss lasting a long time and as another option for foreplay. We'll have an entire section on this due to its notoriety and difficulty level.

- *Sucking:* this form includes sucking her tongue, her lip or nearly any part of her body for a short period. You can suck softly on lips or tongue, or explore a harder sucking feeling and see which one the both of you like best. Sucking can be used for a long duration as well when you are exploring her body – especially good on necks, inner elbows and earlobes.

- *Licking:* often used before actually kissing her, slowly brush across her lip with your tongue. Hold your lips close to her skin and gently lap her skin with a controlled motion of your tongue. This can be quite firm or gentle. Caution needs to be used with this style as well. Some women may be turned off and feel like you're a dog lapping her up.

- *Super sucker:* open your mouth a little more than simply parted and inhale as you kiss her. This will create a vacuum between your mouths and can be a really passionate kiss. Make sure you don't open your mouth too wide or it will be a disaster.

Kisses for Other Parts of the Body

- *Butterfly Kiss:* Use your eyelashes to flutter your girl's lips, nose, neck

- *Necklace Kiss:* Gently kiss or nibble her neck in the shape of a necklace, making sure to get the all-important neck and collarbone. This can be a great warm-up for moving further down, and if you do it slowly and add a little tongue flick into it, she may hurry you along to her breasts.

Kiss Positions

All of these kisses can be done face to face and nose to nose, or you can explore different positions, upside down, rightside up, moving. It's always fun to explore different kissing options with a girl, and when you know the moves, she'll be more confident with you. Also, if you really want to turn her on, make sure to kiss her other sensitive areas, like her collarbone, neck, ears and earlobes, and even the back of the neck.

Amping Up the Kiss – Kissing with Feeling

The difference between a good concert or a bad concert, or a good speech or a bad speech is definitely content and technique. And we've gone over those as far as kissing is concerned. But what really makes a concert, a speech, or a kiss stand out is feeling.

That's why we keep emphasizing going slow, and looking at her. Girls love romance. But the extra special icing on the cake is when you let your feelings show. Not just your 'below the waist' feelings, but your caring, your love.

Now we're not saying that you have to love a girl to kiss her. You probably don't even know her very well. But you do have some feelings for her, and if you are noticing those feelings when you are kissing her, then she'll notice them too and it will be a much better experience.

Timing

Just as there are a lot of methods you can use, timing is crucial for any style you choose. Even the types of kissing can dictate how long you should kiss, when to use the style and when to stop. For example, it's obvious that the peck is used as a quick get-it-over-with type of kiss. The opposite would be the make-out session where the goal is to keep kissing for a long, long time.

Then you have the styles that are in between and could be either short or long depending on the situation.

It's funny, I've found that some girls like to take it slow, kiss for a little while then cuddle, or caress, and some girls like to get really passionate all at once. I love them both! So I try different pacing to find out what she likes. One of the really amazing things I learned doing this is that sometimes if I pull back a little and give her a little space, it turns her on even more, and she'll become more confident and passionate.

Questions you should ask yourself are, "Is this the first time kissing her?" "Does she seem to be enjoying what I'm doing?" "Is this getting boring?" All the questions that you raise should dictate what you do next. Change it up or try a new style to keep things interesting.

Location, Location, Location

If you're just out in the town with your girlfriend and you're being playful and having fun with each other, you may want to use a playful type of kiss and use your imagination to explore different styles. Generally you'll keep these kisses short due to the fact that you're in public.

If you're spending a romantic night at home cuddled on the couch or in front of a fire, this is a great time to go for the more passionate styles. These can range from the sensual, playful and all out French kiss and body kisses of all types. During these moments, the kissing usually is a little more intense and enthusiastic, yet still tender enough that you don't break her neck by being too forceful. Remember to add some feeling to it, and start to notice whether she likes slow or fast – what her pacing is. This will help a lot later on.

CHAPTER 5

Master the French Kiss

Now on to the most famous kiss of all – the French kiss. *Ah, telle est l'amour* (ah, such is love). Just about anyone who has thought about that kiss to end all kisses, the kiss that makes you weak in the knees and the kiss that moves into the bedroom, has declared the French kiss the one that sets your body on fire.

A bit of caution with this somewhat deserved title: this is probably the hardest kiss to pull off and the most dangerous for anyone trying to make an impression. Use it wisely! Don't ever, ever, ever use this kiss until you're sure of her affection for you and the possibility of your relationship moving to the next level. Never use this as a first kiss, no matter what you think might happen next. If you haven't kissed many girls or haven't tried the other styles, definitely skip this one until you've had enough practice to pull it off.

If you're going to attempt this one, there's a few rules you should follow.

First, give it a test. Gently bring your lips to hers, and slip your tongue into the front part of her mouth. See if your tongue meets hers. A great way to get into this kiss is to start with a quick lick of her lips, a taste. If she pulls away from you, stop! She was either taken by surprise or doesn't like the style. Change to a different type of kiss. If she allows it, then swirl your tongue around hers slowly and gently. Try one style for a while, then maybe try some different styles.

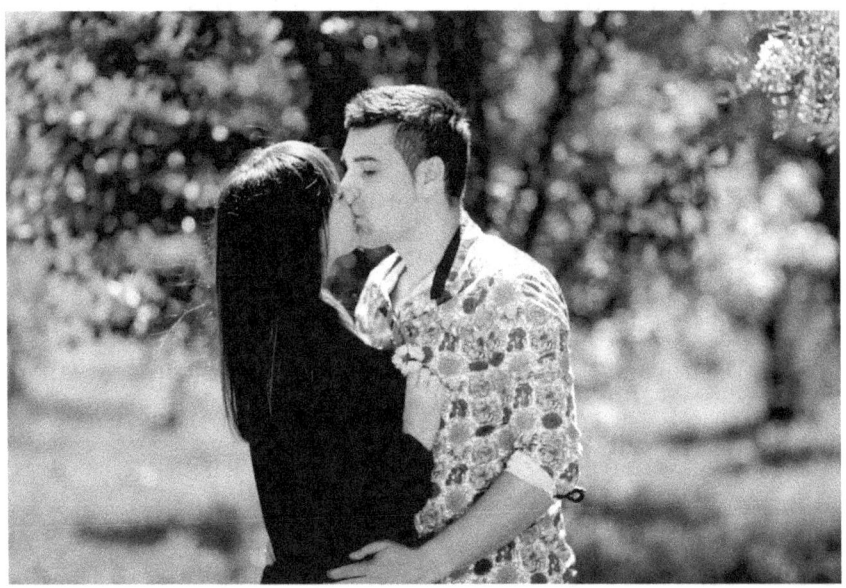

Some variations:

Slow and soft: Let your tongues dance and swirl around each other softly.

Swirl and poke: Add a poke to the swirl, where you press your tongue further into her mouth.

Hard kiss: Put more pressure on your mouth and let your tongue move strongly against hers. This can either really turn her on, or turn her off, so be careful.

Explorer: Run your tongue over her teeth, or the roof of her mouth. Again, best done when you know each other a while.

Finally, don't overdo it! Less is better. That doesn't mean you have to withdraw your tongue immediately, but don't make it last too long. Think of it more as a tease. Let your tongue play with hers for a short time, then go back to your regular kiss. This will make her hot and bothered without turning her off. Not only that, but she'll probably want to come back for more and be more aggressive about it!

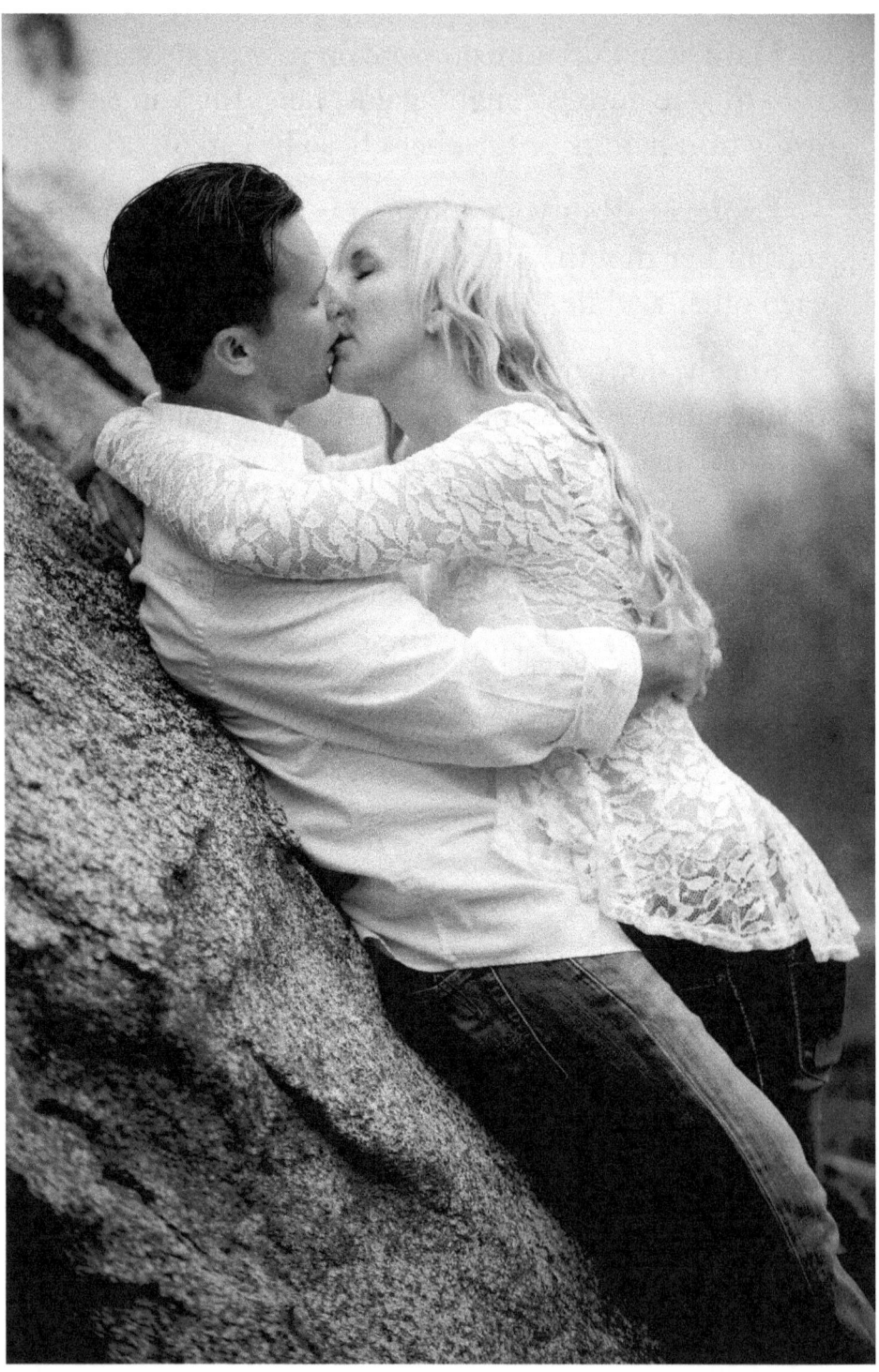

CHAPTER 6

Make It Special: The First Kiss

The first kiss is the kiss that dreams are made of, the one that every man and woman anticipates with excitement and can't wait to talk about. It's also the most important kiss you can ever give a girl, as she will often make up her mind about any further relationship with you based on this one kiss.

Date Prep

Don't forget to use a little preparation. You certainly need to shower before meeting her and use a little cologne or body spray. Make sure your breath smells good by either brushing your teeth or using mouthwash or spray. If you have facial hair, make sure it's groomed well. Also watch out for that stubble! Make sure you shave so you don't scratch her face with yours.

The next important thing is to make yourself more kissable. Yes, there are ways of doing this and the woman

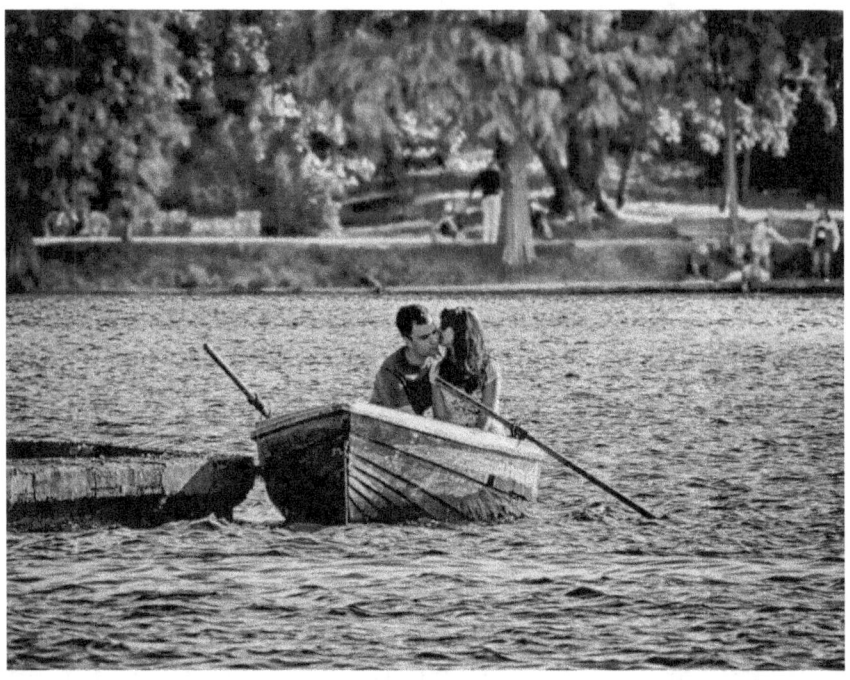

will definitely notice it. First, make sure your lips are looking good. Cracked lips aren't attractive. You want them to be supple and moist. Try using a little Chapstick or balm to keep them looking great.

First Kiss Location

Another important factor for the first kiss is where it occurs. This is even more crucial than with any other type of kiss. Try to think like the woman. She wants it to be perfect with just you and her alone in a nice romantic setting. So, if at all possible, time this kiss when you are in a romantic place, or at least where the ambiance is mood setting. Generally you'll want to be indoors, but if that's not a possibility, try a park or by the water. Sunsets are a perfect time for this kiss no matter what your location. Why? Because women love 'mood' lighting.

Speaking of mood lighting, it's very important indoors as well. If you're at home, set the mood by turning off a few lights or dimming them. Light some candles near the area you'll be together. If you're on a first date and heading out to dinner, be sure to scout the restaurant in advance. Pick one that has the lights set low and candles on the tables. Last, if you have any opportunity to be near a fireplace during the moment, nothing beats the warmth and glow of a fire to really set the mood.

Don't forget her auditory senses too. If you have a chance to play some soft or romantic music, definitely turn it on, but keep it at a low volume. If you don't have music, use your voice. Be sure to chat with her and ask her about herself. You may want to keep your tone soft to create more intimacy between you. Also, don't forget those all-important compliments. Now's the time to give her a few compliments to let her know you really care.

Is She Interested

So you're probably thinking, "How do I know if she will kiss me?" The good news is that she probably wants to be kissed, whether you know it or not. The other good news is she almost undeniably decided within minutes of being with you that she would kiss you. If she's still with you and seems to be enjoying herself, chances are very high that she is hoping you'll kiss her.

There's no tried and true answer to whether or not she wants you to kiss her, but there are definite signs you can look for. First of all, pay attention to what she does. Is she talkative? Does she touch you or hold your hand? These things show she has definite interest in you. One more thing you can look for is if she brushes the hair away from her face with her hand often. Also, if she glances at your lips, that probably means she's thinking about kissing you. Finally, if she leans in towards you, it's a pretty sure sign she's ready for a kiss. It's her way of letting you know it's time for you to make a move.

Pay close attention to her mannerisms. If she doesn't look you in the eye very much or has a closed posture, meaning her arms are crossed or she faces slightly away from you, she may not want to kiss you. Or she could be shy. Watch her lips. If she licks them often or gives them a little nibble once in awhile, she's probably expecting a kiss and it's her way of preparing herself for it.

Another thing to look for is whether she seems to enjoy being with you and likes to keep close or becomes playful with a little nudge or a push. Think of when you were a child and liked a girl. Chances are you did the same type of things to flirt with her. Well, she's doing the exact same thing and it may be the only way she feels comfortable to give you a hint. Sometimes it will come in the form of teasing or joking with you. She wouldn't do any of these things if she didn't have a lot of interest in you.

It's also very important to let her know you are interested in her well before the kiss happens. Make sure you pay a lot of attention to her, listen, listen, listen to what she says. If you're not the best conversationalist, it doesn't matter too much, but if you don't pay attention to her, she'll get the feeling you don't care. That's the worst possible thing you can do during a date.

Compliments go a very long way, but make sure you're being sincere. If you like something about her, say something about her hair, eyes, the way she's dressed, if she's funny or smart – definitely let her know. Flattery will get you everywhere in any situation with a woman as long as you really mean it. However, be careful not to overdo it. A few compliments during the course of an evening is a good rule of thumb.

If you can't think of anything to compliment her on, just tell her you're really enjoying your time with her and you're having fun. Another thing you can try is to touch her gently in appropriate areas like her arm, face, shoulder, etc. Don't do it too often, but once in awhile is a great way to show her you care and you can also see what her reaction is. If she pulls back slightly, it's not the best sign. It doesn't necessarily mean she doesn't like you, it could just be that she's uncomfortable with you touching her until she gets to know you better. Wait a good amount of time and try it again in a different location on her body. Obviously avoid the taboo areas. If she smiles more or becomes more talkative, that's what you're looking for. It means she's receptive to your touch and that she knows you care about her.

Timing

Here's the first place where people go wrong. Most guys think that the first kiss should be at the end of a date. No way. That's way too late. I generally start to warm up to the first kiss about halfway through a date, and make my first move about two-thirds of the way through the date. That way if she takes a little longer to warm up, I have the time, and if she's ready to kiss, we can spend more time getting to know each other that way.

The Approach

Here's the trick, and read this twice. This is how I never get rejected for a kiss. Ever. It's in the approach. By the time my lips are on hers, she's invited me. Here's how it goes.

First off, we're having a good time. If we're not having a good time, then the game's off. Some ways to make sure that she's warming up to you are to ask her questions. Girls love questions. If you just have one question memorized, here it is:

"How did you feel about that?"

It's the question that makes a girl feel close to you. Remember though to ask it about positive or neutral things. Asking her how she felt about her dog dying might bring the whole evening down, and take kissing out of the picture. Ask it about things that happen to her in stories that she tells you about her life.

Compliments are also fantastic. You should mean them, and hopefully if you are out on a date with her, you like something about her! It might be her smile, her hair... make it natural. For example: "I love that necklace – it goes really well with your blue eyes."

Remember, a compliment is always compared to something else, so if you say "Your hair looks great today", then she might take it as "Your hair looks great today compared to how it usually looks." That last one is not so good, so always make the comparison yourself!

The Touch

I always start with the touch. First I'll touch her on the elbow – a very safe place to touch her – and I'll make it look completely natural. For example, I might emphasize a point with a quick (one second) touch to the outside of her elbow. Then I watch to see how she responds. If she moves away, I know to wait a bit. If she moves in or smiles, or looks neutral, I go for another touch.

Good places to touch are her arms and back. I'll also move a little close to her and see if she moves away. This is all getting her warmed up for closer intimacy.

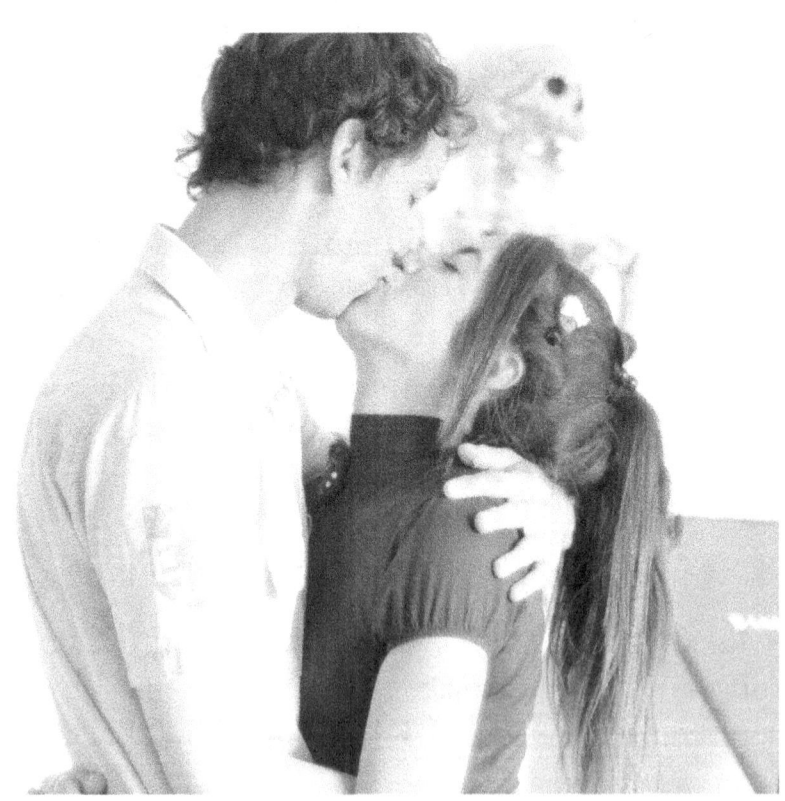

The Kiss

After I've touched her a few times, and she's responded, then I'll casually lean over and touch her hair for a second, and see what she does. I do this in conversation, just as if it is completely natural. If she moves in or smiles, then, a short while later I'll move a bit closer and touch her hair again, for longer, and look at her lips briefly and then into her eyes.

This is almost a non-verbal request to kiss her. If she moves away, or frowns, I move away and wait a little longer, if she moves in or smiles, then she's ready for the kiss. I'm willing to be pretty patient because I've started the whole process about half-way through the date, so I have the rest of the date to get her to the point where we're kissing.

Be confident and don't hesitate. Lean in and hold her gently on the arm, shoulder, neck or small of her back. Women love touch during a kiss and it can make the kiss seem even better than it actually was. A little movement with your hands goes a long way while you kiss her, especially if you move your hand along her neck. It's guaranteed to send shivers down her spine. Remember, how you hold and caress her is just as important, or even more so, as the actual kiss. So much so that it may even be the difference for a not-so-good kiss. If it is a good kiss, it will elevate it to one of the best she ever had.

Now on to the actual kissing. You'll want to slightly part your lips and make it last for a couple to a few seconds. If you feel really confident with the woman, you might also try turning your head slightly to the side either before or during the kiss. This will add a little something special than just the ordinary straight-on kiss. Make sure you close your eyes immediately after your lips touch. This will show her that you're really concentrating on her and are focused on the feeling of the kiss, not how she'll react. It will also put her at ease if she's nervous. Now, if the kiss doesn't seem to go very well, try not to react. Just smile and gaze into her eyes. Nobody can expect a perfect kiss with a new person every time. You haven't kissed each other before, so how could you possibly know how it would work out? You always have another opportunity to try again and get it right the next time. As long as it wasn't a terrible kiss, she'll brush it off and allow you to try again.

CHAPTER 7

Be Irresistible: Bad Kissing vs. Good Kissing

We'll call this the 'rules for kissing. This will help you avoid being a 'bad' kisser and make you more irresistible. Once again, you need to relax and not be concerned too much about kissing. You also need to be confident and don't hesitate.

First let's go over what you should never do. Don't keep your mouth closed unless you're just giving her a peck. At the same time, you don't want to open your mouth too much. For example, your lips should be parted enough to hold a pencil in your mouth, about a quarter of an inch, but no more. If you're trying the sucking style or the French kiss, it's OK to open your mouth a little bit more to allow the technique to work, but definitely don't overdo it. You don't want your mouth to be wide open.

Don't be too aggressive. You shouldn't push your face into hers, only your mouths should touch. Don't hold her too tightly. Women love a gentle touch. It really doesn't matter where you hold her as long as it's not in a 'sexual' area. Once you've been kissing a while you can test out being more aggressive, and see how she likes it. When a woman feels safe with you, sometimes she'll like you being a little more dominant.

Don't use the French kiss until you've tried the other types for a while. If you do try the French kiss, make sure you don't put your tongue in too far, just put it in until her tongue meets yours. Don't dart your tongue in and out repeatedly, this makes for a lousy French kiss. Also, be careful of how 'wet' your mouth is. If you have a lot of moisture, you may want to swallow just before kissing to prevent any excess moisture .

Now on to things you should do. Definitely plan ahead. If you think you might be in a situation where a kiss could occur when meeting your girl, bring your toothbrush and toothpaste with you on the date. Brush your teeth after a meal or drinking. Carry some mouth spray with you. Obviously you shouldn't spray your mouth in front of her before the kiss, so plan for a time where you can do it without her knowing. Try the bathroom just before leaving the restaurant. Ask her to stay in the car so you can open the door for her. Then after you exit the vehicle, give your mouth a couple of sprays. Definitely be gentle, both in the way you hold her and with your kiss. Women love a gentle hug and kiss.

CHAPTER 8

Become a Kissing Master: How to Teach Her to Kiss Better

Whether you're a good kisser or not, you may not like the way SHE kisses. Everybody has their own kissing style and it's common for two different types of kissers to come into conflict. So, what if you don't like what she's doing or you just can't keep up with her style in your own way? Well, that's a sticky situation and it depends on how comfortable you are with her. If you're having your first kissing session and you really like her, don't bring it up just yet. Give it a few tries before attempting to discuss it with her. If you've been dating quite a while or have been in a long relationship, it's something you definitely should bring up.

However, how you bring it up is of utmost importance. The best way to do this is to compliment her on what you do like and ask her if you could kiss like that. Say you want her to slow down or not French kiss so much. Try saying something like this, "I can see you've a very good kisser, but I'm new at this and am having trouble keeping up with you. Could we try and slow it down and keep it simple?" Generally she'll appreciate the compliment and your willingness to be open with her, as long as you use the right approach.

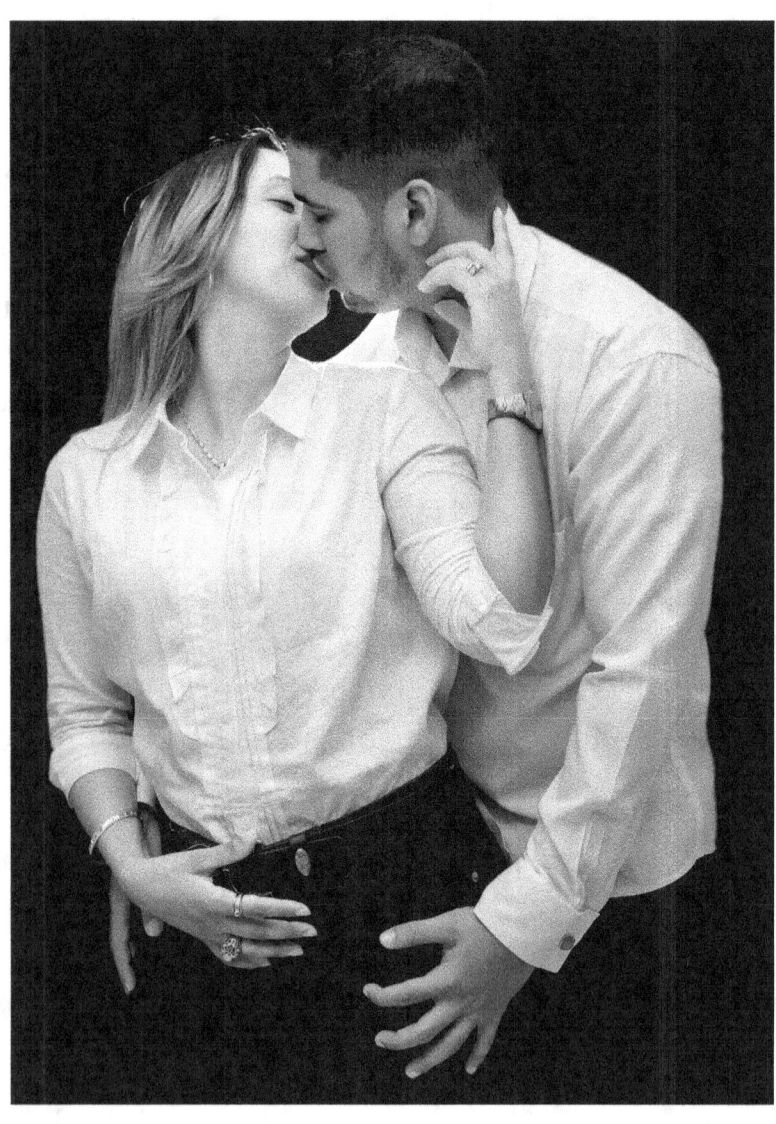

CHAPTER 9

Keep Her Coming Back For More: Advanced Topics

OK, now you've got the kissing thing down and you want to take it to the next level. What do you do now? Well, my dear Watson, trying different styles and altering what you do each time will definitely keep her interested and coming back for more. Teasing her with a couple techniques and changing what you do is the best way to elevate her desire.

The key word is 'tease'. Try a couple of different maneuvers and test them out by keeping them short. See how she reacts. She might move right back in for more, or she might have a confused look on her face. If she comes back for more, change it again and keep her guessing. If she looks confused, try a different style and repeat the process.

Now, this doesn't need to happen in one event, it's better if you try the different styles a little at a time during different situations. Here are a few scenarios you can try out.

The next time you're going to kiss, don't kiss! Yep, it's the ultimate tease and she'll probably love it. Move in and back off a bit, slowly, teasing her to move in closer to you. Just do it once or a couple of times – don't make it last longer than that. After your tease is over, you need to give her the reward. Give her a really good kiss – any style – and make it last a little longer than you normally would.

Next, try just brushing her lips with yours without actually kissing her. Wait until she moves in for the real kiss. The closeness and desire to kiss you will overwhelm her to move in and get it started! Try a combination of the two at the same time. Back off the first time and then just brush her lips the second. However, once you've accomplished the 'tease' and she moves in for the real thing, meet her lips and give her the kiss she really wants.

Try a different amount of pressure. Maybe start gently and then push your face in to hers a little to make it into something 'hotter'. Again, don't push too hard, but a little more than usual.

Another thing you can try is to gently suck on her lip – top or bottom – and then give her a little nibble. After that, back off and see what she does. You may want to try that without backing off and go back to kissing normally. Then try a little French kiss when things are heating up. Put your tongue in and swirl it around hers just once, then go back to whatever you were doing. She might come back for more French kissing or let you continue to stay in control.

Last, don't forget other parts of her face and neck. If things are really going well, try gently nibbling on her earlobe or bring your kiss down to her chin and neck. If she's in the mood for this, you'll have her begging for more. Again, just give her a teaser for a little while when kissing her in different places, then move back to her mouth.

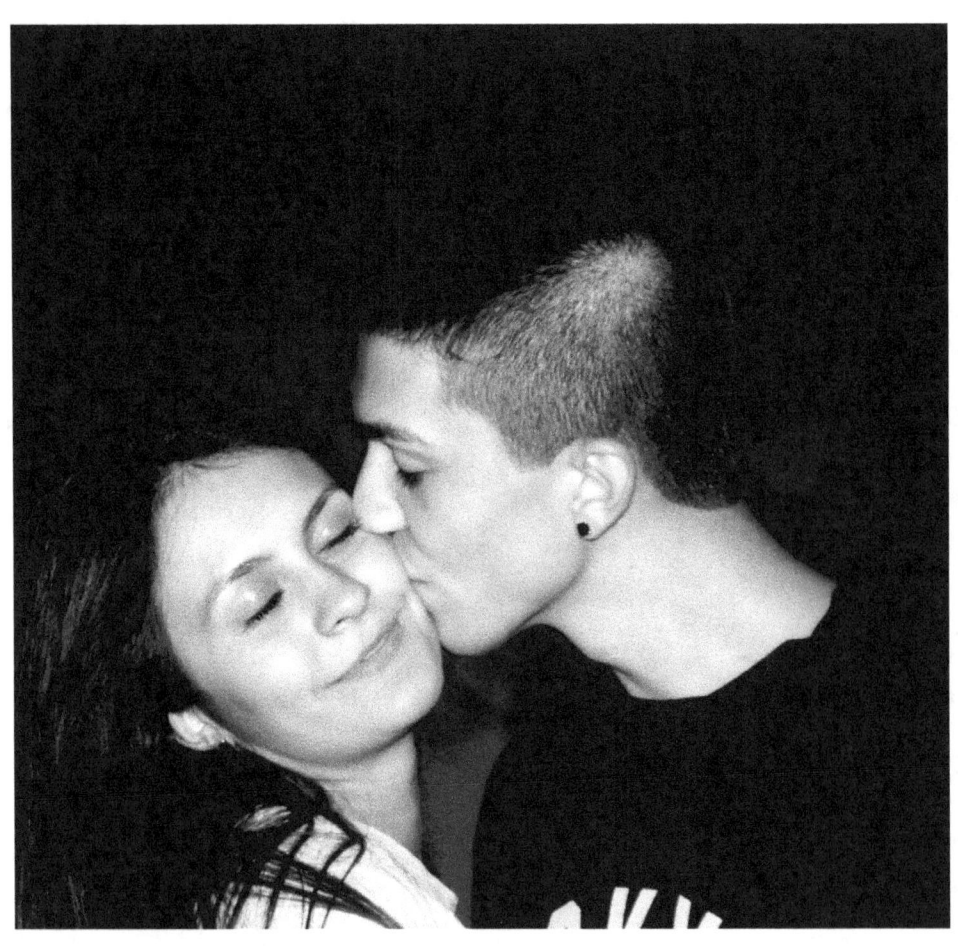

CHAPTER 10

Your Questions Answered

Now it's time to answer the most commonly asked questions related to kissing. Below is a Q&A of most of the questions you might have. We hope it helps to give you the last bit of information, and confidence, you need.

Q: How do I kiss with braces?

A: There are absolutely no reasons why braces should prevent you from kissing. If you both wear braces, the likelihood of them somehow getting caught on each other is extremely low. Not only that, but you shouldn't be concerned about whether she thinks her or your braces aren't attractive enough to kiss, because they're not a problem. Many people with braces actually say they've been kissed more with them then when they didn't have them. So, forget about it, it's not even an issue.

Q: Is gay, lesbian or transgendered kissing any different?

A: Absolutely not. If you're not heterosexual, don't even be concerned. Everything in this guide is meant for everyone, no matter what your sexual orientation. However, if you have any question as to whether the other person has the same orientation as you, don't attempt to kiss them until you're absolutely sure.

Q: What kind of kissing do women like?

A: Most like all of the types listed in this report, with the possible exception of the French kiss, particularly when you're just getting to know each other. That's why you need to be very cautious before and during the use of this style. Otherwise, try them all out, we're sure you will keep her guessing and find out what works best for the two of you.

Q: Should you kiss her?

A: The best thing is to go with your gut instinct. If it's telling you not to kiss her, there's probably a reason for it. Wait a bit longer and see if your feelings change. Chances are she wants to be kissed if things are going well between you. Watch for the telltale signs – her touching you, brushing the hair away from her face, when she leans in toward you, etc.

Q: When is the best time to kiss?

A: There's no real answer for this question. Anytime is a good time. However, you definitely want to wait at least an hour or two if you're out on a first date. Whenever it 'feels' right and you seem to be pretty close, that's the best time to give it a try, no matter when or where you are. You don't necessarily need to wait until a date is at the end. The only other hangup some women may have is showing their affection in public. This doesn't mean you shouldn't try to kiss her when in public, but definitely pay attention to her reaction. If it doesn't go well and she pulls back or keeps it short, then you probably should avoid it.

Q: Does it feel different when you kiss different people?

A: A definite yes. Everyone has their own style and feelings about one another. You may have a 'bad' kisser on one date and the next one will knock your socks off. There's no way to determine if someone is a 'bad' or 'good' kisser until you actually kiss. Once you find someone who knocks your socks off, you'll definitely want to have a lot more of where that came from.

Q: What is a kiss and why is it so desirable?

A: A kiss can be any style and placed anywhere on the body. As long as it involves your lips touching another person, it's considered a kiss. Science has tried to find proof of why kisses are so desirable, but there's little evidence that points to anything specific. It's definitely something most people enjoy because it shows affection, love, care and closeness. It's also well known to lead to other more intimate moments.

Q: How should I practice kissing?

A: There are many ways you can practice before landing that smooch on your significant other. One of the best methods is to practice on a pillow. It's close enough to kissing a real face and gives you a chance to practice how you plan to hold the woman at the same time. Try kissing your hand or arm too. Obviously it's skin so it makes for a good surface to practice on. Also, you'll be able to feel what she will feel as far as your lips meeting hers.

CHAPTER 11

Top 10 Tips for Great Kisses

1. *Make it private.* Face it, you can kiss her anywhere, but to really give her what she needs, privacy is the best option. That way neither you nor her have to worry about others watching or being interrupted. Not only that, but it's a heck of a lot easier to be in complete focus on each other and really 'feel' the pleasure. It may also lead to a lot more and she'll be open to exploration if it's just the two of you.

2. *Take it easy.* Definitely don't rush it. Slow and gentle is better. Also, don't let it last too long. Not only will you avoid turning her off by staying in the kiss for too long, chances are she'll enjoy it more and keep coming back for the same feeling.

3. *Compliment and caress.* Nothing turns a woman on or makes her more receptive to you than compliments and touch. Again, be sure you are sincere when complimenting her. The best bets are to talk about her eyes, hair or her dress. That's exactly

what she wants to hear and she'll definitely feel better about you and be more willing to enjoy the kiss. Also, a gentle touch now and then works wonders. Start with simple touches, like on her arm, elbow, shoulder or face. Then increase your caressing leading up to your kiss. You'll definitely put her in the mood and prepare her for what's coming next.

4. *Tease, tease, tease!* If you've got her where you want her, moving in slowly and not kissing her can turn her on as much as the kiss itself. When you do kiss, make it short and pull back a little, then go in for more. Try teasing her lips by rubbing your mouth against them without actually kissing her. Nibble on her lip a little, then go back to kissing. These methods are virtually guaranteed to drive her wild.

5. *Slow is key.* Remember, a kiss doesn't have to start with a kiss. Try nuzzling her a little on her neck or cheek. Whisper sweet nothings in her ear. This will definitely get her more aroused and ready for your next play. The more time you spend caressing and tantalizing her mind, the more she'll be anticipating the kiss and be more receptive when you actually kiss her.

6. *Be a little more aggressive.* Again, the key here is a little! Try putting your hand on the back of her neck and add a little more pressure to your kiss.

This will definitely turn her on and give her a real idea of what you want to do next. Then move to her ear and give her a little suck on her lobe. After that, move down to her neck and spend a good amount of time there, kissing her all over. Once you move back up to her mouth, it's virtually guaranteed she'll be ready and waiting for that ultimate kiss to come.

7. *Add a little body maneuver.* Try giving her a little dip if you feel comfortable and strong enough to do so. If not, try slowly laying her down on a couch or bed. This will take your kiss to the next level. If you don't feel comfortable using this technique then move in close and hold her firmly against your body. The more surface your bodies touch, the more passionate the kiss will be.

8. *Rub a dub dub.* Caressing her all over will elevate her feelings and put her on top of the world. Move your hands up and down her back and arms. Caress her face and hair. Just be sure to use a gentle touch to really turn her on.

9. *Use variety.* Kissing the same way all the time can get a little monotonous. Start kissing one way, then quickly change to another style. Take quick breaks and hit her with another style she isn't expecting. This will keep her guessing and throw her off balance, exactly what you need to keep her attention piqued.

10. *Go for it all!* If all the above is working, time to move on to bigger and better things. Now it's time to move your hands to her nether regions and get her gasping for air. The best bet is to start with a gentle squeeze on her buttocks and move along her legs. If you really want to heat things up, move your hands to her inner thighs or near her breasts, without touching them. If she's receptive, it'll drive her crazy that you're so close to her major erogenous zones and won't be able to wait for you to get right to them.

CHAPTER 12

Summing It All Up

The key to remember is relax and be confident, or at least appear to be confident! Don't let your nerves take a hold of you. Move with purpose and be gentle. As long as you remember this and act accordingly, she won't know that you haven't done this before or aren't sure of yourself. You may not have done it before and you may not be sure, but the only thing you need to worry about is what SHE thinks. As long as she doesn't suspect a thing, you have nothing to worry about.

Just remember that this isn't rocket science and millions of people have come before you without any real problems. Everybody has to have a first kiss and everybody needs to do it a few times to get it perfect. Think of it as riding a bike. You didn't just get on and take off down the street without falling unless someone held on to you while you made your attempt. However, after a few tries, your body took over and learned how to balance just right without thinking much about it. It's the same with kissing, you have her to hold onto and you may not be Don Juan the first time you make the attempt. Neither will she and she needs you as much as you need her during the big moment.

If you read this entire guide, you have as much as you need to make your first kiss, or to kiss your significant other better than ever before. The only step you need to take is to try different things and some of the more advanced information to become the ultimate kisser. Once you have the basics down, you'll need to explore the other methods on your own to get to where you want to be. Don't be afraid to experiment and use the advice in this book. The only way you'll get better is to be open to new techniques and change it up a little every so often.

Whatever you do from here on out, don't waste what you learned. Take the advice we gave you and use it. Why not, it certainly can't hurt and can only make you a better kisser! If you choose not to, not only have you wasted your time, you definitely won't become the ultimate kissing machine that every woman will swoon over. So, don't just toss this information aside and forget it, there's a reason why you read this and it's a very good one.

Don't let your effort go to waste. We assure you that if you follow the advice, you will be much better off than you were before you read this. We're not saying you need to try everything you've read. You may totally disagree with one or more of the kissing styles because it just isn't 'you'. That's absolutely fine, but don't miss out on all the other goodies you have read.

Think about it this way – if you wanted to learn how to fix the plumbing under your sink, would you just read a little bit and then toss the information out and forget it? We hope not, because that would probably end in a disaster with your house flooding, or you'd need to hire a professional to finish what you started. You wouldn't hire a professional kisser to handle your woman for you, would you? So, take this advice and become the professional yourself. It's the only way you'll ever become the best kisser a woman could ever ask for!

Finally, the best advice you can follow from this report is to always pay attention to the woman. We've brought it up numerous times throughout the guide to make sure you understand its importance. Ignoring any of it will surely lead you on a path to nowhere. Remember, it's the little things that mean the most when it comes to women. She won't make anything obvious for you and will expect you to still get the message, so pay attention.

Mannerisms can be the hardest thing to decipher and take a long time to understand. It's like taking an exam sometimes. You've done your homework and it's still grueling to get through the entire test with a good grade. It takes a lot of time and patience to master. Unfortunately, it can sometimes take a couple of years for some men to finally discover what a woman means by her actions. Some of us pick up on them easily and become masters quickly. You know those men because they always seem to have a woman with them and plenty more lined up to take over when the opportunity presents itself. You may have always thought it was because they're good looking, rich, a star or just popular. Yes, all of these things help you attract a woman, but keeping her and making her happy requires something more than just who you are.

Have you ever seen an ugly guy with a gorgeous woman? Why do you think that happened? You probably brush it off by proclaiming he must be rich or some other means of dismissing the relationship as just a fluke. Well, chances are he pays a lot of attention to the woman and really understands how she works. It's a lot harder for a man to be with someone he's not attracted to, but for a woman it's not always about looks, she wants someone she can really be in love with and who gives her the attention that will really light her up.

So, now that you know that it isn't just the kiss that means the world to a woman, that it's really what leads up to the kiss that actually matters, now it's time for you to start utilizing what you have learned and start your journey to becoming a master kisser. Finally, it's time for you to study her, mimic her at times, get to the root of what she's saying to you in a nonverbal manner.

Listen to her, pay attention to her, touch her, be close

to her. Use every opportunity she gives you to learn more about what she's trying to tell you. Watch her movements closely: in her face, in her hand gestures, the way she touches you and her posture. If she's giving you signals that say 'come hither', make sure you respond by moving in a little closer. If she touches you, return the favor. If she likes to hug a lot, be sure to give her a hug before kissing her. No matter how she acts, as long as you pay attention and respond to what she's doing, you'll be that much closer to making her happy and fulfilling her desires. Follow these simple rules and we guarantee that you'll enjoy a much fuller love life than you ever have before.

www.ingramcontent.com/pod-product-compliance
Lightning Source LLC
Chambersburg PA
CBHW070128290526
45789CB00005B/2160